CHEMO-FRIENDLY MEALS:
Nourishing Recipes for Cancer Patients

By Yuri G Allman

INTRODUCTION

Nutrition plays a critical role in supporting the body during chemotherapy treatment. "Chemo Friendly Meals" is a comprehensive guide designed to help individuals undergoing chemotherapy to plan and prepare meals that are both delicious and nutritious. The book covers everything from the importance of nutrition during chemotherapy, to tips for meal planning and recommended food groups and nutrient-rich foods. It also includes a variety of easy-to-prepare recipes for breakfast, lunch, dinner, and snacks that are specifically tailored to support the body during chemotherapy. This book will empower you to take control of your nutrition during this challenging time and provide your body with the essential nutrients it needs to fight against cancer. Whether you're the patient or a caregiver, this book is a valuable resource that will help you to support your loved one during chemotherapy journey

CONTENT

WHAT ARE CHEMO-FRIENDLY MEALS?

Chemo-friendly meals are foods that are easy to digest and are gentle on the stomach for individuals undergoing chemotherapy treatment. These meals are often high in protein and calories to help maintain weight and strength, and low in fat and fiber to reduce discomfort and diarrhea. Examples of chemo-friendly meals include broths, soups, cooked vegetables, fruits, and lean proteins such as chicken, fish, and eggs. Individuals undergoing chemotherapy should consult with their healthcare provider or a dietitian for specific recommendations.

In addition to being easy to digest and high in protein, chemo-friendly meals should also be well-cooked and soft in texture. This can include baked or steamed fish, soft-boiled eggs, cooked vegetables, and pureed fruits. It is also important to stay hydrated while undergoing chemotherapy, so drinking plenty of water, clear broths, and other fluids can help. Some individuals may also benefit from taking a liquid supplement to help meet their nutritional needs.

It is important to note that everyone's body reacts differently to chemotherapy, so what may be tolerated by one person may not be for another. It is important to pay attention to one's own body and how it reacts to different foods.

It is also important to be mindful of food safety and hygiene during and after chemotherapy as the treatment can weaken the immune system. This can include avoiding raw or undercooked foods, and practicing good hygiene while handling and preparing food.

IMPORTANCE OF NUTRITION DURING CHEMOTHERAPY

Nutrition plays a critical role during chemotherapy as it can help to maintain strength, prevent infection and support the healing process. During chemotherapy, the body's metabolism can change, leading to weight loss, fatigue and muscle wasting. Adequate nutrition can help to prevent these complications and support the body's ability to fight off infection.

Protein is especially important during chemotherapy as it is essential for building and repairing body tissues, and maintaining a healthy immune system. Carbohydrates are also important as they provide energy for the body. Additionally, foods high in vitamins and minerals, such as fruits and vegetables, can help to support the body's overall health and well-being.

Maintaining a healthy weight is also important during chemotherapy as it can help to prevent fatigue and support the body's ability to fight off infection. Eating a balanced diet that is high in protein and calories can help to maintain weight and muscle mass.

In summary, maintaining a healthy diet during chemotherapy is essential for providing the body with the nutrients it needs to fight off infection, heal, and maintain strength and energy levels. It is important for the person undergoing chemotherapy to work with a healthcare professional to develop a suitable nutrition plan.

TIPS FOR MEAL PLANNING DURING CHEMOTHERAPY

Consult with a registered dietitian or a healthcare provider to develop a personalized nutrition plan that meets your specific needs.

Plan for small, frequent meals throughout the day rather than large meals. This can help to reduce nausea and make it easier to consume enough calories and nutrients.

Include high-protein foods in your diet such as lean meats, fish, eggs, dairy, and legumes.

Include foods high in vitamins and minerals, such as fruits and vegetables.

Choose well-cooked, soft foods that are easy to digest, such as baked or steamed fish, soft-boiled eggs, cooked vegetables, and pureed fruits.

Stay hydrated by drinking plenty of water and clear fluids.

Prepare meals and snacks in advance and store them in the refrigerator or freezer for easy access when needed.

Avoid foods that are high in fat, fiber, or spicy flavors, as they can cause stomach discomfort.

Be mindful of food safety and hygiene during and after chemotherapy as the treatment can weaken the immune system.

Be flexible and willing to try new foods and recipes. Some foods that you used to enjoy may not be appealing during chemotherapy, so it is important to be open to trying new things.

RECOMMENDED FOOD GROUPS AND NUTRIENT-RICH FOODS

During chemotherapy, it is important to consume a variety of nutrient-rich foods from different food groups to ensure that the body is getting all the necessary vitamins, minerals and other nutrients. Here are some recommended food groups and nutrient-rich foods that can be included in a chemo-friendly diet:

Protein:

Lean meats such as chicken, turkey, and fish
Eggs
Dairy products such as milk, yogurt, and cheese
Legumes such as beans, lentils, and peas
Tofu

Carbohydrates:

Whole grains such as bread, rice, and pasta
Starchy vegetables such as potatoes, sweet potatoes, and corn
Fruits such as berries, apples, and bananas

Fruits and Vegetables:

Leafy greens such as spinach, kale, and broccoli
Orange and yellow fruits and vegetables, such as sweet potatoes, carrots, and squash
Berries and citrus fruits like oranges, lemons, and limes

Vitamins and Minerals:

Foods high in vitamin C, such as oranges, lemons, limes, kiwi, and strawberries, help to support the immune system
Foods high in vitamin A, such as sweet potatoes, carrots, and squash, which are important for the health of the eyes and skin.
Foods high in zinc, such as oysters, beef, and fortified cereals, which are important for the immune system and wound healing

Foods high in iron, such as red meat, poultry, and leafy greens, which are important for maintaining healthy red blood cells.

BREAKFAST

1 Scrambled Eggs with Cooked Vegetables:

Ingredients:

2 eggs
1/4 cup diced spinach
1/4 cup diced mushrooms
Salt and pepper, to taste
1 tsp butter or oil

Instructions:

Heat a small skillet over medium heat. Add the butter or oil.
Once the butter or oil is hot, add the diced spinach and mushrooms. Cook for 2-3 minutes until softened.
In a small bowl, beat the eggs with a fork.
Season with salt and pepper.

Pour the beaten eggs over the vegetables in the skillet and stir gently with a spatula until the eggs are cooked through, about 2-3 minutes. Serve hot.

2 Greek Yogurt with Berries and a Drizzle of Honey:

Ingredients:

1 cup Greek yogurt
1/2 cup mixed berries (such as strawberries, blueberries, and raspberries)
1 tbsp honey

Instructions:

In a small bowl, mix together the Greek yogurt and honey.
In a separate bowl, mix together the mixed berries.
Serve the yogurt mixture with the mixed berries on top and drizzle with honey.

3 Cream of Rice Cereal with Milk and Chopped Nuts:

Ingredients:

1/2 cup cooked cream of rice cereal
1/2 cup milk
2 tbsp chopped nuts (such as almonds or walnuts)

Instructions:

Cook cream of rice cereal according to package instructions.
In a small bowl, mix together the cooked cream of rice cereal and milk.
Top with chopped nuts.

4 Soft-Boiled Eggs with Toast and Butter:

Ingredients:

2 eggs
2 slices of toast

1 tbsp butter

Instructions:

Place eggs in a saucepan and cover with water.
Bring the water to a boil.
Once the water is boiling, let the eggs cook for
4-5 minutes.
Remove the eggs from the water and cool
slightly.
Toast the bread slices and spread butter on top.
Peel the eggs and serve on top of toast.

5 Omelet with Cheese and Herbs:

Ingredients:

2 eggs
1/4 cup shredded cheese (such as cheddar or
mozzarella)
1 tbsp chopped herbs (such as parsley or chives)
Salt and pepper, to taste
1 tsp butter or oil

Instructions:

In a small bowl, beat the eggs with a fork. Add the shredded cheese, herbs, salt and pepper.
Heat a small skillet over medium heat. Add the butter or oil.
Pour the egg mixture into the skillet and cook for 2-3 minutes, until the bottom is set.
Carefully fold the omelette in half and cook for an additional 1-2 minutes, until the cheese is melted.
Serve hot.

6 Smoothie made with Yogurt, Fruit, and Honey:

Ingredients:

1 cup Greek yogurt
1/2 cup mixed berries (such as strawberries, blueberries, and raspberries)
1/2 banana
1 tbsp honey

Instructions:

Add the Greek yogurt, mixed berries, banana and honey to a blender.
Blend until smooth.
Serve immediately.

7 Avocado Toast with a Fried Egg:

Ingredients:

1 avocado
2 slices of bread
Salt and pepper, to taste
1 egg
1 tsp butter or oil

Instructions:

Toast the bread slices.
In a small bowl, mash the avocado with a fork and season with salt and pepper.
Spread the mashed avocado on top of the toast slices.

Heat a small skillet over medium heat. Add the butter or oil.

Once the butter or oil is hot, crack the egg into the skillet and cook for 2-3 minutes, until the whites are set and the yolk is cooked to your preference.

Place the fried egg on top of the avocado toast. Serve immediately.

8 French Toast made with Soft Bread and Served with Syrup:

Ingredients:

2 eggs
1/4 cup milk
2 slices of soft bread
1 tbsp butter
Maple syrup, for serving

Instructions:

In a shallow dish, whisk together the eggs and milk.

Dip the slices of bread in the egg mixture, making sure to coat both sides.
Heat a skillet over medium heat. Add the butter. Once the butter is melted, add the bread slices to the skillet. Cook for 2-3 minutes per side, until golden brown.
Serve with maple syrup.

9 Yogurt Parfait with Granola, Yogurt, and Fruit:

Ingredients:

1 cup Greek yogurt
1/4 cup granola
1/4 cup mixed berries (such as strawberries, blueberries, and raspberries)

Instructions:

In a small bowl, mix together the Greek yogurt and granola.
In a separate bowl, mix together the mixed berries.

Layer the yogurt mixture and mixed berries in a cup or glass. Repeat until the cup or glass is filled.
Serve immediately.

10 Soft Scrambled Eggs with Cheese and Herbs:

Ingredients:

2 eggs
1/4 cup shredded cheese (such as cheddar or mozzarella)
1 tbsp chopped herbs (such as parsley or chives)
Salt and pepper, to taste
1 tsp butter or oil

Instructions:

In a small bowl, beat the eggs with a fork. Add the shredded cheese, herbs, salt and pepper.
Heat a small skillet over medium heat. Add the butter or oil.
Pour the egg mixture into the skillet and cook, stirring gently with a spatula, until the eggs are

cooked through and the cheese is melted, about
2-3 minutes.
Serve hot.

11 Creamy Oatmeal with Milk and Honey:

Ingredients:

1/2 cup rolled oats
1 cup milk
1 tbsp honey

Instructions:

Cook oatmeal according to package instructions.
In a small bowl, mix together the cooked
oatmeal and milk.
Stir in honey.
Serve hot.

12 Breakfast Burrito with Scrambled Eggs, Cheese, and Avocado:

Ingredients:

2 eggs
1/4 cup shredded cheese (such as cheddar or mozzarella)
1 avocado
2 tortillas
Salt and pepper, to taste
1 tsp butter or oil

Instructions:

In a small bowl, beat the eggs with a fork.
Season with salt and pepper.
Heat a small skillet over medium heat. Add the butter or oil.
Pour the beaten eggs into the skillet and cook, stirring gently with a spatula,
until the eggs are cooked through and the cheese is melted, about 2-3 minutes.
4. In a separate small bowl, mash the avocado with a fork. Season with salt and pepper.
Warm the tortillas in the microwave or on a skillet.

Place the scrambled eggs and mashed avocado on the center of each tortilla.
Roll the tortilla around the filling, tucking in the sides to make a burrito.
Serve immediately.

13 Quiche with a Soft Crust and Cooked Vegetables:

Ingredients:

2 eggs
1/4 cup milk
1/4 cup diced cooked vegetables (such as spinach, mushrooms, bell peppers)
1/4 cup shredded cheese (such as cheddar or mozzarella)
Salt and pepper, to taste
1 pre-made pie crust or homemade crust

Instructions:

Preheat the oven to 350°F (175°C).
In a small bowl, beat the eggs and milk together.

Mix in the diced vegetables, shredded cheese, salt and pepper.

Pour the mixture into the pie crust.

Bake for 25-30 minutes, or until the center is set and the crust is golden brown.

Let cool slightly before slicing and serving.

14 Muffins made with Soft Fruits, such as Banana or Berries:

Ingredients:

1 cup all-purpose flour
1 tsp baking powder
1/4 tsp salt
1/2 cup mashed banana or mixed berries
1/2 cup sugar
1 egg
1/2 cup milk

Instructions:

Preheat the oven to 350°F (175°C).

In a medium bowl, mix together the flour, baking powder, and salt.
In a separate bowl, mix together the mashed banana or mixed berries, sugar, egg, and milk.
Add the wet ingredients to the dry ingredients and mix until just combined.
Pour the batter into a muffin tin, filling each cup about 2/3 of the way full.
Bake for 18-20 minutes, or until a toothpick inserted into the center comes out clean.
Let cool before serving.

15 Breakfast Sandwich with Scrambled Eggs, Cheese, and Bacon:

Ingredients:

2 eggs
1/4 cup shredded cheese (such as cheddar or mozzarella)
2 slices of bacon
2 slices of bread
1 tsp butter or oil

Instructions:

In a small bowl, beat the eggs with a fork.
Season with salt and pepper.
Heat a small skillet over medium heat. Add the
butter or oil.
Pour the beaten eggs into the skillet and cook,
stirring gently with a spatula, until the eggs are
cooked through and the cheese is melted, about
2-3 minutes.
Cook the bacon in a separate skillet until crispy.
Toast the bread slices.
Assemble the sandwich by placing the
scrambled eggs and bacon on one slice of toast
and topping with the other slice of toast.
Serve immediately.

16 Breakfast Casserole with Eggs, Cheese, and
Cooked Vegetables:

Ingredients:

6 eggs
1/2 cup milk

1/2 cup shredded cheese (such as cheddar or
mozzarella)
1/2 cup diced cooked vegetables (such as
spinach, mushrooms, bell peppers)
Salt and pepper, to taste

Instructions

Preheat the oven to 350°F (175°C).
In a large bowl, beat the eggs and milk together.
Mix in the shredded cheese, diced vegetables,
salt, and pepper.
Pour the mixture into a greased 9x13 inch
baking dish.
Bake for 25-30 minutes, or until the center is set
and the top is golden brown.
Let cool slightly before serving.

17 Breakfast Smoothie Bowl with Yogurt,
Frozen Fruit, and Granola:

Ingredients:

1 cup Greek yogurt

1/2 cup frozen mixed berries (such as strawberries, blueberries, and raspberries)
1/2 banana
1 tbsp honey
1/4 cup granola

Instructions:

Add the Greek yogurt, frozen mixed berries, banana and honey to a blender.
Blend until smooth.
Pour the smoothie into a bowl and top with granola.
Serve immediately.

18 Soft Boiled Eggs with Toast Soldiers:

Ingredients:

2 eggs
4 slices of bread (cut into thin strips)
Butter, for spreading

Instructions:

Place eggs in a saucepan and cover with water.
Bring the water to a boil.
Once the water is boiling, let the eggs cook for
4-5 minutes.
Remove the eggs from the water and cool
slightly.
Toast the bread strips and spread butter on top.
Peel the eggs and serve with the toast strips.

19 Creamy Polenta with Milk, Butter, and
Cheese:

Ingredients:

1 cup polenta
4 cups water
1/4 cup milk
1 tbsp butter
1/4 cup shredded cheese (such as cheddar or
mozzarella)
Salt and pepper, to taste

Instructions:

Bring 4 cups of water to a boil in a medium saucepan.
Slowly stir in the polenta and continue to stir for 2-3 minutes, until the polenta thickens.
Remove from heat, and stir in the milk, butter, cheese, salt, and pepper.
Serve hot.

20 Scrambled Eggs with Diced Cooked Ham and Cheese:

Ingredients:

2 eggs
1/4 cup diced cooked ham
1/4 cup shredded cheese (such as cheddar or mozzarella)
Salt and pepper, to taste
1 tsp butter or oil

Instructions:

In a small bowl, beat the eggs with a fork.
Season with salt and pepper.
Heat a small skillet over medium heat. Add the
butter or oil.
Once the butter or oil is hot, add the diced
cooked ham and cook for 1-2 minutes.
Pour the beaten eggs over the cooked ham in the
skillet and stir gently with a spatula until the
eggs are cooked through, about 2-3 minutes.
Stir in shredded cheese and cook until melted.
Serve hot.
All of these recipes are chemo friendly, as they
are easily digestible, and do not contain any
ingredients that could be harmful to someone
undergoing chemotherapy.

LUNCH

1 Grilled Chicken or Fish with Cooked
Vegetables:

Marinate chicken or fish in a mixture of olive
oil, lemon juice, and herbs of your choice (such
as parsley, thyme, and rosemary) for at least 30
minutes.
Heat a grill or grill pan over medium-high heat.
Grill the chicken or fish for 4-5 minutes per side,
or until cooked through.
Steam or boil asparagus or green beans for 3-4
minutes, or until tender.
Serve the grilled chicken or fish with the cooked
vegetables on the side.

2 Creamy Tomato Soup with a Grilled Cheese
Sandwich:

In a large pot, sauté diced onions and garlic in
butter or olive oil until softened.

Add canned crushed tomatoes and chicken or vegetable broth. Bring the mixture to a boil, then reduce the heat and simmer for 10-15 minutes. Use an immersion blender to blend the soup until smooth. Stir in heavy cream and season with salt and pepper to taste.

For the sandwich, butter two slices of bread and place a slice of cheese between them. Grill in a pan or on a sandwich press until the bread is golden brown and the cheese is melted.

Serve the soup with the grilled cheese sandwich on the side.

3 Turkey and Cheese Sandwich on Soft White Bread:

Spread mayonnaise or mustard on one side of two slices of white bread.

Top one slice with sliced turkey and cheese, and the other slice with lettuce and tomato.

Press the two slices together to make a sandwich.

Cut the sandwich in half and serve.

4 Baked Salmon with a Side of Cooked Rice:

Preheat the oven to 400 degrees F.
Place a piece of salmon on a baking sheet lined with parchment paper.
Drizzle olive oil over the salmon and season with salt, pepper and herbs of your choice.
Bake for 10-15 minutes, or until the salmon is cooked through.
Cook rice according to package instructions.
Serve the baked salmon with the cooked rice on the side.

5 Minestrone Soup with a Side of Crackers or Bread:

In a large pot, sauté diced onions, carrots, and celery in olive oil until softened.
Add canned diced tomatoes, vegetable broth, and your choice of vegetables such as green beans, zucchini, and kidney beans. Bring the

mixture to a boil, then reduce the heat and simmer for 20-25 minutes.
Season with salt, pepper, and herbs of your choice.
Serve the soup with crackers or bread on the side.

6 Chicken or Turkey Salad with Lettuce and Tomato on a Soft Roll:

In a large bowl, mix shredded chicken or turkey with mayonnaise, chopped celery, and herbs of your choice.
Season with salt and pepper to taste.
Spread the chicken or turkey salad on the roll and top with lettuce and tomato.
Serve.

7 Creamy Macaroni and Cheese with Cooked Vegetables:

Cook macaroni according to package instructions.

In a separate pot, melt butter and whisk in flour to make a roux. Slowly add milk, stirring constantly, until the mixture thickens. Stir in shredded cheese until melted.

Add the cooked macaroni to the cheese sauce and stir to combine.

Steam or boil vegetables of your choice (such as broccoli or carrots) for 3-4 minutes, or until tender.

Serve the macaroni and cheese with the cooked vegetables on the side.

8 Vegetable Soup with a Side of Soft Bread:

In a large pot, sauté diced onions, carrots, and celery in olive oil until softened.

Add canned diced tomatoes, vegetable broth, and your choice of vegetables such as spinach, zucchini, and potatoes. Bring the mixture to a boil, then reduce the heat and simmer for 20-25 minutes.

Season with salt, pepper, and herbs of your choice.
Serve the soup with soft bread on the side.

9 Baked Chicken with a Side of Mashed Potatoes:

Preheat the oven to 400 degrees F.
Place chicken breasts on a baking sheet lined with parchment paper.
Drizzle olive oil over the chicken and season with salt, pepper, and herbs of your choice.
Bake for 20-25 minutes, or until the chicken is cooked through.
Peel and boil potatoes until tender, then mash them with butter, milk, and seasonings of your choice.
Serve the baked chicken with the mashed potatoes on the side.

10 Egg Salad Sandwich on Soft White Bread:

Boil eggs, cool them and peel off the shell.
In a large bowl, mash the eggs with mayonnaise, chopped celery, and herbs of your choice.
Season with salt and pepper to taste.
Spread the egg salad on one slice of bread and top with lettuce.
Place the other slice of bread on top to make a sandwich.
Cut the sandwich in half and serve.

11 Grilled Cheese Sandwich with Tomato and Basil:

Butter two slices of bread and place a slice of cheese between them.
Add sliced tomato and basil leaves, then press the two slices together to make a sandwich.
Grill the sandwich in a pan or on a sandwich press until the bread is golden brown and the cheese is melted.
Cut the sandwich in half and serve.

12 Tuna Salad Sandwich on Soft White Bread:

In a large bowl, mix canned tuna with mayonnaise, chopped celery, and herbs of your choice.
Season with salt and pepper to taste.
Spread the tuna salad on one slice of bread and top with lettuce.
Place the other slice of bread on top to make a sandwich.
Cut the sandwich in half and serve.

13 Chicken or Turkey and Vegetable Stir-Fry with Rice:

Cook rice according to package instructions.
In a large pan or wok, heat oil over high heat.
Add diced chicken or turkey and stir-fry for 3-4 minutes, or until cooked through.
Add your choice of vegetables such as bell peppers, carrots, and snow peas. Stir-fry for an additional 2-3 minutes, or until the vegetables are tender.

Season the stir-fry with soy sauce and herbs of your choice.
Serve the stir-fry with the cooked rice on the side.

14 Cream of Broccoli Soup with a Side of Crackers or Bread:

In a large pot, sauté diced onions and garlic in butter or olive oil until softened.
Add chopped broccoli florets and chicken or vegetable broth. Bring the mixture to a boil, then reduce the heat and simmer for 10-15 minutes, or until the broccoli is tender.
Use an immersion blender to blend the soup until smooth. Stir in heavy cream and season with salt and pepper to taste.
Serve the soup with crackers or bread on the side.

15 Grilled Chicken with a Side of Quinoa:

Cook quinoa according to package instructions. Marinate chicken in a mixture of olive oil, lemon juice, and herbs of your choice (such as parsley, thyme, and rosemary) for at least 30 minutes. Heat a grill or grill pan over medium-high heat. Grill the chicken for 4-5 minutes per side, or until cooked through.
Serve the grilled chicken with the cooked quinoa on the side.

16 Lentil Soup with a Side of Soft Bread:

In a large pot, sauté diced onions, carrots, and celery in olive oil until softened.
Add canned diced tomatoes, vegetable broth, and lentils. Bring the mixture to a boil, then reduce the heat and simmer for 20-25 minutes.
Season with salt, pepper, and herbs of your choice.
Serve the soup with soft bread on the side.

17 Broiled Fish with a Side of Cooked Potatoes:

Preheat the broiler to high heat.

Place a piece of fish on a baking sheet lined with foil.

Drizzle olive oil over the fish and season with salt, pepper, and herbs of your choice.

Broil for 5-7 minutes per side, or until the fish is cooked through.

Peel and boil potatoes until tender, then mash them with butter, milk, and seasonings of your choice.

Serve the broiled fish with the cooked potatoes on the side.

18 Cream of Mushroom Soup with a Side of Crackers or Bread:

In a large pot, sauté diced onions and garlic in butter or olive oil until softened.

Add sliced mushrooms, chicken or vegetable broth, and herbs of your choice. Bring the mixture to a boil, then reduce the heat and simmer for 10-15 minutes.

Use an immersion blender to blend the soup until smooth. Stir in heavy cream and season with salt and pepper to taste.
Serve the soup with crackers or bread on the side.

19 Baked Chicken with a Side of Cooked Pasta:

Preheat the oven to 400 degrees F.
Place chicken breasts on a baking sheet lined with parchment paper.
Drizzle olive oil over the chicken and season with salt, pepper, and herbs of your choice.
Bake for 20-25 minutes, or until the chicken is cooked through.
Cook pasta according to package instructions.
Serve the baked chicken with the cooked pasta on the side.

20 Chicken or Turkey and Cheese Wrap with Lettuce and Tomato:

Spread mayonnaise or mustard on a large flour tortilla.

Place shredded chicken or turkey, cheese, lettuce and tomato on the tortilla.

Roll up the tortilla to make a wrap.

Cut the wrap in half and serve.

DINNER

1 Grilled Chicken or Fish with Cooked Vegetables:

Ingredients:

4 boneless, skinless chicken breasts or 4 fish
fillets (such as salmon or tilapia)
2 tbsp olive oil
Salt and pepper, to taste
1 lb asparagus or green beans, trimmed

Instructions:

Preheat your grill to medium-high heat.
Brush the chicken or fish with olive oil and
season with salt and pepper.
Grill the chicken or fish for about 4-5 minutes
per side, or until cooked through.
Meanwhile, bring a pot of salted water to a boil.
Add the asparagus or green beans and cook for
2-3 minutes, or until tender.
Drain the vegetables and season with salt and
pepper.
Serve the chicken or fish with the cooked
vegetables.

2 Creamy Chicken or Vegetable Risotto:

Ingredients:

2 tbsp butter
1 onion, diced
2 cloves of garlic, minced
1 cup Arborio rice
3 cups chicken or vegetable broth
1 cup heavy cream
1 cup grated Parmesan cheese
1 cup diced cooked chicken or vegetables
(optional)

Instructions:

In a large pot or Dutch oven, melt the butter over
medium heat.
Add the onion and garlic and cook until
softened.
Add the rice and stir to coat in the butter.
Slowly add the broth, one ladleful at a time,
stirring constantly.

Wait until the liquid is absorbed before adding the next ladleful.
Once the rice is cooked through and creamy, stir in the heavy cream and Parmesan cheese.
If using, stir in the diced chicken or vegetables.
Serve the risotto hot.

3 Baked Salmon with a Side of Cooked Rice:

Ingredients:

4 salmon fillets
2 tbsp olive oil
Salt and pepper, to taste
2 cups water
1 cup white or brown rice

Instructions:

Preheat your oven to 375°F (190°C).
Place the salmon fillets in a baking dish and brush with olive oil.
Season with salt and pepper.

Bake the salmon for 12-15 minutes, or until cooked through.

Meanwhile, bring the water to a boil in a medium saucepan.

Add the rice, reduce the heat to low, and cover.

Cook for 18-20 minutes, or until the water is absorbed.

Fluff the rice with a fork and season with salt and pepper.

Serve the baked salmon with the cooked rice.

4 Minestrone Soup with a Side of Crackers or Bread:

Ingredients:

2 tbsp olive oil
1 onion, diced
2 cloves of garlic, minced
2 carrots, diced
2 celery stalks, diced
1 can diced tomatoes
4 cups chicken or vegetable broth
1 can kidney beans, rinsed and drained

1 cup uncooked small pasta, such as ditalini
Salt and pepper, to taste

5 Crackers or bread, for serving

Instructions:

In a large pot or Dutch oven, heat the olive oil
over medium heat.
Add the onion, garlic, carrots, and celery and
cook until softened.
Stir in the diced tomatoes, broth, kidney beans,
and pasta.
Bring the soup to a boil, then reduce the heat and
simmer for 20-25 minutes, or until the pasta is
cooked through.
5. Season the soup with salt and pepper to taste.
Serve the minestrone soup with crackers or
bread on the side.

5 Chicken or Turkey Stew with Vegetables and
Potatoes:

Ingredients:

2 tbsp olive oil

1 onion, diced

2 cloves of garlic, minced

2 cups diced cooked chicken or turkey

2 cups diced potatoes

2 cups diced carrots

1 cup frozen peas

2 cups chicken or vegetable broth

1 tsp dried thyme

Salt and pepper, to taste

Instructions:

In a large pot or Dutch oven, heat the olive oil over medium heat.

Add the onion and garlic and cook until softened.

Stir in the chicken or turkey, potatoes, carrots, and frozen peas.

Pour in the broth and add the thyme, salt and pepper.

Bring the stew to a boil, then reduce the heat and simmer for 20-25 minutes, or until the vegetables are tender.
Serve the stew hot.

6 Creamy Macaroni and Cheese with Cooked Vegetables:

Ingredients:

8 oz uncooked elbow macaroni
2 tbsp butter
2 tbsp flour
2 cups milk
1 cup grated cheddar cheese
Salt and pepper, to taste
1 cup cooked vegetables (such as broccoli or peas)

Instructions:

Cook the macaroni according to package instructions. Drain and set aside.

In a large saucepan, melt the butter over medium heat.
Stir in the flour to make a roux.
Slowly pour in the milk, stirring constantly.
Cook until the mixture thickens.
Stir in the cheddar cheese until melted.
Season the cheese sauce with salt and pepper.
Stir in the cooked macaroni and vegetables.
Serve the macaroni and cheese hot.

7 Vegetable Soup with a Side of Soft Bread:

Ingredients:

2 tbsp olive oil
1 onion, diced
2 cloves of garlic, minced
2 cups diced carrots
2 cups diced potatoes
2 cups frozen mixed vegetables
4 cups chicken or vegetable broth
Salt and pepper, to taste
Soft bread, for serving

Instructions:

In a large pot or Dutch oven, heat the olive oil over medium heat.
Add the onion and garlic and cook until softened.
Stir in the carrots, potatoes, mixed vegetables and broth.
Bring the soup to a boil, then reduce the heat and simmer for 20-25 minutes, or until the vegetables are tender.
Season the soup with salt and pepper to taste.
Serve the soup hot with soft bread on the side.

8 Baked Chicken with a Side of Mashed Potatoes:

Ingredients:

4 boneless, skinless chicken breasts
2 tbsp olive oil
Salt and pepper, to taste
2 cups water

1 lb potatoes, peeled and diced
1/4 cup milk or cream
2 tbsp butter

Instructions:

Preheat your oven to 375°F (190°C).
Place the chicken breasts in a baking dish and brush with olive oil.
Season with salt and pepper.
Bake the chicken for 25-30 minutes, or until cooked through.
Meanwhile, bring the water to a boil in a medium saucepan.
Add the potatoes, reduce the heat to low, and cover.
Cook for 15-20 minutes, or until the potatoes are tender.
Drain the potatoes and mash them with milk or cream and butter.
Season with salt and pepper to taste.
Serve the baked chicken with the mashed potatoes.

9 Egg Salad Sandwich on Soft White Bread:

Ingredients:

6 boiled eggs, peeled and diced
2 tbsp mayonnaise
1 tbsp Dijon mustard
Salt and pepper, to taste
Lettuce leaves, for serving
Soft white bread, for serving

Instructions:

In a medium bowl, combine the diced eggs, mayonnaise, Dijon mustard, salt and pepper.
Mix well.
Spread the egg salad mixture on a slice of soft white bread.
Add lettuce leaves and sandwich it with another slice of bread.
Serve the sandwich immediately.

10 Grilled Cheese Sandwich with Tomato and Basil:

Ingredients:

4 slices of white or wheat bread
4 slices of cheddar cheese
2 tbsp butter
2-3 slices of tomato
Fresh basil leaves, for serving

Instructions:

Preheat a skillet over medium heat.
Place a slice of cheese between two slices of bread.
Spread butter on one side of the sandwich.
Place the sandwich in the skillet, butter side down.
Repeat with the remaining sandwiches.
Cook the sandwiches for 2-3 minutes on each side, or until the bread is golden brown and the cheese is melted.
Slice the sandwiches in half and serve with the tomato slices and basil leaves.

11 Tuna Salad Sandwich on Soft White Bread:

Ingredients:

1 can of drained tuna
2 tbsp mayonnaise
1 tbsp Dijon mustard
Salt and pepper, to taste
Lettuce leaves, for serving
Soft white bread, for serving

Instructions:

In a medium bowl, combine the tuna,
mayonnaise, Dijon mustard, salt and pepper.
Mix well.
Spread the tuna salad mixture on a slice of soft
white bread.
Add lettuce leaves and sandwich it with another
slice of bread.
Serve the sandwich immediately.

12 Chicken or Turkey and Vegetable Stir-Fry with Rice:

Ingredients:

2 tbsp vegetable oil
1 onion, diced
2 cloves of garlic, minced
2 cups diced cooked chicken or turkey
2 cups diced vegetables (such as bell peppers, broccoli, or carrots)
2 cups cooked white or brown rice
2 tbsp soy sauce
1 tsp sesame oil
Salt and pepper, to taste

Instructions:

Heat the oil in a large skillet or wok over high heat.
2. Add the onion and garlic and stir-fry for 1-2 minutes.

Add the chicken or turkey and vegetables and continue to stir-fry for an additional 2-3 minutes, or until the vegetables are tender.

Stir in the cooked rice, soy sauce, and sesame oil.
Season with salt and pepper to taste.
Serve the stir-fry hot.

13 Cream of Broccoli Soup with a Side of Crackers or Bread:

Ingredients:

2 tbsp butter
1 onion, diced
2 cloves of garlic, minced
2 cups diced broccoli florets
4 cups chicken or vegetable broth
1 cup heavy cream
Salt and pepper, to taste
Crackers or bread, for serving

Instructions:

In a large pot or Dutch oven, melt the butter over medium heat.

Add the onion and garlic and cook until softened.

Stir in the broccoli and broth.

Bring the soup to a boil, then reduce the heat and simmer for 15-20 minutes, or until the broccoli is tender.

Carefully puree the soup in a blender or use an immersion blender until smooth.

Stir in the heavy cream and season with salt and pepper to taste.

Serve the soup hot with crackers or bread on the side.

14 Grilled Chicken with a Side of Quinoa:

Ingredients:

4 boneless, skinless chicken breasts
2 tbsp olive oil
Salt and pepper, to taste
2 cups water
1 cup quinoa

Instructions:

Preheat your grill to medium-high heat.
Brush the chicken with olive oil and season with salt and pepper.
Grill the chicken for about 4-5 minutes per side, or until cooked through.
Meanwhile, bring the water to a boil in a medium saucepan.
Add the quinoa, reduce the heat to low, and cover.
Cook for 18-20 minutes, or until the water is absorbed.
Fluff the quinoa with a fork and season with salt and pepper.
Serve the grilled chicken with the quinoa.

15 Lentil Soup with a Side of Soft Bread:

Ingredients:

2 tbsp olive oil
1 onion, diced
2 cloves of garlic, minced
1 cup lentils, rinsed and drained

4 cups chicken or vegetable broth
1 can diced tomatoes
Salt and pepper, to taste
Soft bread, for serving

Instructions:

In a large pot or Dutch oven, heat the olive oil over medium heat.
Add the onion and garlic and cook until softened.
Stir in the lentils, broth, and diced tomatoes.
Bring the soup to a boil, then reduce the heat and simmer for 25-30 minutes, or until the lentils are tender.
Season the soup with salt and pepper to taste.
Serve the soup hot with soft bread on the side.

16 Broiled Fish with a Side of Cooked Potatoes:

Ingredients:

4 fish fillets (such as salmon or tilapia)
2 tbsp olive oil

Salt and pepper, to taste
2 cups water
1 lb potatoes, peeled and diced

Instructions:

Preheat your broiler to high heat.
Place the fish fillets on a broiler pan and brush with olive oil.
3. Season with salt and pepper.
Broil the fish for about 4-5 minutes per side, or until cooked through.
Meanwhile, bring the water to a boil in a medium saucepan.
Add the potatoes, reduce the heat to low, and cover.
Cook for 15-20 minutes, or until the potatoes are tender.
Drain the potatoes and season with salt and pepper to taste.
Serve the broiled fish with the cooked potatoes.

17 Cream of Mushroom Soup with a Side of Crackers or Bread:

Ingredients:

2 tbsp butter
1 onion, diced
2 cloves of garlic, minced
2 cups sliced mushrooms
4 cups chicken or vegetable broth
1 cup heavy cream
Salt and pepper, to taste
Crackers or bread, for serving

Instructions:

In a large pot or Dutch oven, melt the butter over medium heat.
Add the onion and garlic and cook until softened.
Stir in the mushrooms and broth.
Bring the soup to a boil, then reduce the heat and simmer for 15-20 minutes, or until the mushrooms are tender.
Carefully puree the soup in a blender or use an immersion blender until smooth.

Stir in the heavy cream and season with salt and pepper to taste.
Serve the soup hot with crackers or bread on the side.

17 Baked Chicken with a Side of Cooked Pasta:

Ingredients:

4 boneless, skinless chicken breasts
2 tbsp olive oil
Salt and pepper, to taste
8 oz uncooked pasta (such as spaghetti or fettuccine)

Instructions:

Preheat your oven to 375°F (190°C).
Place the chicken breasts in a baking dish and brush with olive oil.
Season with salt and pepper.
Bake the chicken for 25-30 minutes, or until cooked through.
Meanwhile, bring a pot of salted water to a boil.

Add the pasta and cook according to package instructions.
Drain the pasta and season with salt and pepper to taste.
Serve the baked chicken with the cooked pasta.

18 Chicken or Turkey and Cheese Wrap with Lettuce and Tomato:

Ingredients:

2 cups diced cooked chicken or turkey
1/2 cup grated cheese (such as cheddar or Monterey jack)
2 tbsp mayonnaise
1 tbsp Dijon mustard
Salt and pepper, to taste
Lettuce leaves
Sliced tomatoes
Flour or corn tortillas

Instructions:

In a medium bowl, combine the chicken or turkey, cheese, mayonnaise, Dijon mustard, salt and pepper.
Mix well.
Place some of the mixture on a tortilla.
Add lettuce leaves, tomatoes and wrap it.
Repeat with the remaining mixture and tortillas.
Serve the wraps immediately.

19 Cream of Potato Soup with a Side of Crackers or Bread:

Ingredients:

2 tbsp butter
1 onion, diced
2 cloves of garlic, minced
2 cups diced potatoes
4 cups chicken or vegetable broth
1 cup heavy cream
Salt and pepper, to taste
Crackers or bread, for serving

Instructions:

In a large pot or Dutch oven, melt the butter over medium heat.

2. Add the onion and garlic and cook until softened.

Stir in the potatoes and broth.

Bring the soup to a boil, then reduce the heat and simmer for 15-20 minutes, or until the potatoes are tender.

Carefully puree the soup in a blender or use an immersion blender until smooth.

Stir in the heavy cream and season with salt and pepper to taste.

Serve the soup hot with crackers or bread on the side.

20 Baked salmon with a lemon and herb topping:

Ingredients:

4 salmon fillets

1 lemon, juiced
2 cloves of garlic, minced
2 tablespoons of olive oil
1 teaspoon of dried thyme
1 teaspoon of dried basil
Salt and pepper, to taste

Instructions:

Preheat your oven to 375 degrees F (190 degrees C).

In a small bowl, mix together the lemon juice, garlic, olive oil, thyme, basil, salt, and pepper.

Place the salmon fillets on a baking sheet lined with foil or parchment paper.

Brush the lemon and herb mixture over the top of the salmon.

Bake the salmon in the preheated oven for 15-20 minutes, or until the fish is cooked through and flakes easily with a fork.

Serve and enjoy!

CHEMO FRIENDLY ENTREES AND SIDES WITH RECIPES

1 Baked Salmon with Lemon and Herbs:

4 salmon fillets
2 tablespoons olive oil
Salt and pepper to taste
2 cloves of minced garlic
2 tablespoons of fresh lemon juice
2 tablespoons of chopped fresh herbs (such as dill, parsley, or basil)

Instructions:

Preheat the oven to 400 degrees F.

Line a baking sheet with parchment paper.

Place the salmon fillets on the baking sheet.

In a small bowl, mix together the olive oil, garlic, lemon juice, salt, and pepper.

Brush the mixture over the salmon fillets.

Sprinkle the chopped herbs over the fillets.

Bake for 12-15 minutes, or until the fish is cooked through.

2 Creamy Chicken and Vegetable Risotto:

1 tablespoon olive oil
1 onion, chopped
2 cloves of minced garlic
1 cup of Arborio rice
3 cups of chicken broth
1 cup of diced cooked chicken
1 cup of diced cooked vegetables (such as asparagus, mushrooms, or peas)
1/2 cup of grated Parmesan cheese
Salt and pepper to taste

Instructions:

In a large skillet, heat the olive oil over medium heat.

Add the onion and garlic and cook until softened.

Add the rice and stir to coat it with the oil.

Slowly add the chicken broth, stirring constantly.

Cook, stirring occasionally, until the rice is cooked and the mixture is creamy.

Stir in the chicken and vegetables, and cook until heated through.

Stir in the Parmesan cheese and season with salt and pepper to taste.

3 Cream of Broccoli Soup:

2 tablespoons of butter
1 onion, chopped

2 cloves of minced garlic

4 cups of broccoli florets

4 cups of chicken or vegetable broth

1 cup of milk or cream

Salt and pepper to taste

Instructions:

In a large pot, melt the butter over medium heat.

Add the onion and garlic and cook until softened.

Add the broccoli and broth, and bring to a simmer.

Cook for about 10 minutes or until the broccoli is tender.

Use an immersion blender or carefully transfer the soup to a blender and puree until smooth.

Return the soup to the pot and stir in the milk or cream.

Season with salt and pepper to taste.

4 Grilled Vegetable and Quinoa Salad:

1/2 cup of quinoa
1 cup of water or chicken broth
Salt and pepper to taste
1 teaspoon olive oil
1 red bell pepper, sliced
1 yellow bell pepper, sliced
1 zucchini, sliced
1 red onion, sliced
1/4 cup of chopped fresh herbs (such as parsley, basil, or mint)
2 tablespoons of lemon juice

Instructions:

Rinse the quinoa in a fine-mesh strainer.
In a medium saucepan, bring the quinoa, water or broth, and a pinch of salt to a boil.
Reduce the heat and simmer, covered, for about 15 minutes or until the quinoa is tender.

Remove from heat and let sit for 5 minutes.
Fluff with a fork.
Preheat grill to medium-high heat.

In a large bowl, toss the vegetables with the olive oil, salt, and pepper.

Grill the vegetables for about 5-7 minutes per side, or until tender and charred.

In a large bowl, combine the quinoa, grilled vegetables, herbs, and lemon juice.

Season with salt and pepper to taste.

5 Creamy Potato Soup:

2 tablespoons of butter
1 onion, chopped
2 cloves of minced garlic
4 cups of diced potatoes
4 cups of chicken or vegetable broth
1 cup of milk or cream
Salt and pepper to taste

Instructions:

In a large pot, melt the butter over medium heat.

Add the onion and garlic and cook until softened.

Add the potatoes and broth, and bring to a simmer.

Cook for about 15 minutes or until the potatoes are tender.

Use an immersion blender or carefully transfer the soup to a blender and puree until smooth.

Return the soup to the pot and stir in the milk or cream.

Season with salt and pepper to taste.

6 Baked Chicken with Herbs:

4 chicken breasts
2 tablespoons of olive oil
Salt and pepper to taste
2 cloves of minced garlic
2 tablespoons of chopped fresh herbs (such as thyme, rosemary, or oregano)

Instructions:

Preheat the oven to 400 degrees F.

Line a baking sheet with parchment paper.

Place the chicken breasts on the baking sheet.

In a small bowl, mix together the olive oil, garlic, salt, and pepper.

Brush the mixture over the chicken breasts.

Sprinkle the chopped herbs over the chicken.

Bake for 25-30 minutes, or until the chicken is cooked through.

7 Grilled Chicken and Vegetable Skewers:

1 pound of boneless, skinless chicken breasts, cut into cubes
1 red bell pepper, cut into chunks
1 yellow bell pepper, cut into chunks
1 red onion, cut into chunks
2 tablespoons of olive oil
Salt and pepper to taste
2 cloves of minced garlic
2 tablespoons of chopped fresh herbs (such as parsley, basil, or mint)

Instructions:

Preheat grill to medium-high heat.

In a large bowl, toss the chicken, bell peppers, and onion with the olive oil, salt, pepper, garlic, and herbs.

Thread the chicken and vegetables onto skewers.

Grill the skewers for about 8-10 minutes per side, or until the chicken is cooked through and the vegetables are tender.

8 Creamy Pasta with Vegetables:

8 ounces of pasta (such as fettuccine, penne, or rigatoni)
2 tablespoons of butter
1 onion, chopped
2 cloves of minced garlic
1 cup of diced cooked vegetables (such as asparagus, mushrooms, or peas)
1/2 cup of heavy cream
1/2 cup of grated Parmesan cheese
Salt and pepper to taste

Instructions:

Cook the pasta according to package instructions.
In a large skillet, melt the butter over medium heat.

Add the onion and garlic and cook until softened.
Add the vegetables and cook until tender.
Stir in the cream and Parmesan cheese, and cook until the sauce

is heated through and the cheese is melted.
6. Add the cooked pasta to the skillet and toss to coat it with the sauce.

Season with salt and pepper to taste.

9 Vegetable and Tofu Stir Fry:

1 tablespoon of vegetable oil
1 onion, chopped
2 cloves of minced garlic
1 cup of diced cooked vegetables (such as bell peppers, carrots, and broccoli)
1 cup of diced firm tofu
2 tablespoons of soy sauce
1 tablespoon of rice vinegar
1 teaspoon of corn starch
Salt and pepper to taste

Instructions:

In a large skillet or wok, heat the oil over medium-high heat.

Add the onion and garlic and cook until softened.

Add the vegetables and tofu, and cook until the vegetables are tender.

In a small bowl, mix together the soy sauce, rice vinegar, corn starch, salt, and pepper.

Pour the mixture over the stir-fry and toss to coat the vegetables and tofu.

Cook for another minute or until the sauce thickens.

10 Creamy Polenta with Parmesan and Herbs:

4 cups of water

Salt and pepper to taste
1 cup of polenta
1/2 cup of grated Parmesan cheese
2 tablespoons of butter
2 tablespoons of chopped fresh herbs (such as parsley, basil, or mint)

Instructions:

In a medium saucepan, bring the water to a boil and season with salt.
Slowly whisk in the polenta and reduce the heat to low.
Cook for about 15-20 minutes or until the polenta is tender.

Remove from heat and stir in the Parmesan cheese, butter, and herbs.
5. Season with salt and pepper to taste.

CHEMO FRIENDLY SMOOTHIES

1 Berry Bliss Smoothie:

Blend 1 cup frozen berries, 1 banana, 1/2 cup Greek yogurt, and 1/2 cup almond milk.

2 Ginger-Turmeric Smoothie:

Blend 1 banana, 1/2 cup frozen pineapple, 1/2 inch ginger root, 1/4 teaspoon turmeric, 1/2 cup coconut milk, and 1/2 cup ice.

3 Green Machine Smoothie:

Blend 1 banana, 1/2 avocado, 1 cup spinach, 1/2 cup Greek yogurt, and 1/2 cup almond milk.

4 Peach-Mango Smoothie:

Blend 1 peach, 1/2 cup frozen mango, 1/2 banana, 1/2 cup Greek yogurt, and 1/2 cup orange juice.

5 Carrot-Orange Smoothie:

Blend 1 carrot, 1 orange, 1/2 banana, 1/2 cup Greek yogurt, and 1/2 cup almond milk.

6 Chocolate-Avocado Smoothie:

Blend 1 avocado, 1 banana, 1/4 cup cocoa powder, 1/2 cup Greek yogurt, and 1/2 cup almond milk.

7 Apple-Cinnamon Smoothie:

Blend 1 apple, 1 banana, 1/2 teaspoon cinnamon, 1/2 cup Greek yogurt, and 1/2 cup almond milk.

8 Lemon-Coconut Smoothie:

Blend 1/2 cup coconut milk, 1/2 cup Greek yogurt, 1/2 banana, 1/4 cup frozen pineapple, 1 teaspoon honey, 1/2 teaspoon lemon zest.

9 Pumpkin-Spice Smoothie:

Blend 1/2 cup pumpkin puree, 1 banana, 1/2 teaspoon pumpkin pie spice, 1/2 cup Greek yogurt, and 1/2 cup almond milk.

10 Strawberry-Banana Smoothie:

Blend 1 cup frozen strawberries, 1 banana, 1/2 cup Greek yogurt, and 1/2 cup almond milk.

Note: Avoid ingredients that may cause gastric irritation and check with your doctor or dietitian before consuming them during chemotherapy.

CHEMO FRIENDLY SNACKS RECIPES

1 Greek Yogurt with Berries:

Top 1/2 cup Greek yogurt with a mixture of fresh or frozen berries.

2 Hummus with Vegetables:

Dip sliced cucumber, bell peppers, or carrot sticks in 1/4 cup hummus.

3 Baked Sweet Potato:

Bake a sweet potato and top with butter and a sprinkle of cinnamon.

4 Hard-Boiled Eggs:

Boil and peel eggs for a quick and easy high-protein snack.

5 Avocado Toast:

Mash half an avocado onto a piece of whole-grain toast and sprinkle with salt and pepper.

6 Cottage Cheese with Fruit:

Top 1/2 cup cottage cheese with your favorite fresh or canned fruit.

7 Chocolate-Dipped Frozen Banana:

Peel and freeze a banana, then dip in melted dark chocolate.

8 Smoothie with Spinach:

Blend 1/2 cup Greek yogurt, 1/2 cup frozen berries, 1 banana, and 1 cup spinach for a nutrient-rich snack.

9 Apple Slices with Peanut Butter:

Spread peanut butter on slices of apple for a healthy and satisfying snack.

10 Frozen Grapes:

Rinse and freeze grapes for a sweet and refreshing snack.

Printed in Great Britain
by Amazon

26098907R00056